Home Office Wellness Guide

Ergonomic Habits For A Healthier, More Productive Workday

Dr. Susan Jameson, Chiropractor

Better Back Solutions

Home Office Wellness Guide – Ergonomic Habits For A Healthier, More Productive Workday

This book is intended for informational purposes only. It is not a substitute for professional medical advice, diagnosis, or treatment. Always consult with a qualified healthcare provider before making any changes to your healthcare or ergonomic setup.

Author: Dr. Susan Jameson, Chiropractor

Title: Home Office Wellness Guide

Subtitle: Ergonomic Habits For A Healthier, More Productive Workday

First Edition: 2025

Print ISBN: 978-1-7640830-2-7

Published by: Better Back Solutions

National Library of Australia

Cataloging-in-Publication entry available upon request. Legal deposit compliant with the Copyright Act1968 (Cth).

Praise For Home Office Wellness Guide

"Just what I needed to address daily fatigue while working at home and in the office."

"Practical, easy-to-follow guidance that turns good intentions into real habits."

"Clear, detailed methods that explain not just what to do — but why it works."

"Helped me improve my energy, mood, and productivity throughout the day."

"A comprehensive, well-organised guide covering ergonomics, movement, hydration, sleep, and focus."

"Managing energy, not hours, finally made sense."

— Readers

Introduction

From Comfort to Vitality: The Next Step in Ergonomic Living

The way we work has changed forever. Home offices, flexible schedules, and hybrid teams are now a normal part of professional life — but so too are the hidden strains that come with long hours at a screen. Many people have learned how to make their workspace comfortable; fewer have learned how to make it *energizing*.

This book was created to fill that gap.

In my first book, *Home Office Handbook - Ergonomic Solutions for Back Pain*, I focused on helping readers create safe, supportive workspaces that reduce musculoskeletal strain. That guide explored posture alignment, chair setup, and workstation design — the *physical foundations* of pain-free work.

This new volume, *Home Office Wellness Guide: Ergonomic Habits for a Healthier, More Productive Workday*, builds upon those principles and takes them further. Here, we move beyond the physical setup and explore **how daily habits, movement, light, hydration, and recovery influence focus, energy, and long-term wellbeing.**

The goal is not perfection — it's *awareness and rhythm*. You'll learn how to integrate small, restorative actions into the flow of your day: how to move more naturally, manage energy cycles, reduce digital overload, and create a workspace that supports both productivity and calm.

Each chapter offers practical steps grounded in science and experience. You'll find tools for movement and posture, ways to protect your eyes and wrists, insights into circadian rhythms and light exposure, and strategies to balance focus with recovery. Together, these form a modern wellness system for remote and hybrid professionals — one that supports mind, body, and work performance in equal measure.

The workplace has shifted from buildings to bodies — from where we work to *how* we work.
Your home office can be more than a desk; it can be a place of energy, comfort, and renewal.

Let this guide help you design that experience — one mindful habit at a time.

How To Use This Book

Turning Knowledge Into Daily Wellness

This guide is designed to be practical — something you can apply in real time, not just read and set aside. Each chapter builds on the last, moving from physical comfort to energy management and emotional wellbeing.

You don't need to read it all at once. You can move through it sequentially, or dip into the chapters that best fit your current needs — whether it's improving focus, reducing fatigue, or creating better digital boundaries.

Along the way, you'll find:

• Science-based explanations that connect ergonomics to energy, focus, and health
• Simple daily habits — posture resets, movement breaks, and mindfulness techniques — you can begin immediately
• Reflection prompts and action plans to help turn new insights into lasting habits

If you've already read *Home Office Handbook – Ergonomic Solutions for Back Pain*, consider that book your foundation for physical setup. This guide builds upon it, focusing on habits, rhythm, and resilience rather than equipment alone.

You may also find the *Home Office Journal – A 30-Day Ergonomic Workbook* helpful for putting these principles into daily practice.

Your workspace can become a place of restoration as well as productivity. Let's begin.

Table of Contents

CHAPTER 1

THE NEW WORK LANDSCAPE

How Hybrid and Remote Work Reshaped the Way We Live, Move, and Recover

The modern workplace has shifted dramatically. What was once a clear divide between office and home has blurred into a single, always-connected environment. For millions of professionals, the home office is now the center of productivity — but also, increasingly, a source of physical strain, digital fatigue, and emotional overload.

Remote and hybrid work have brought undeniable benefits: flexibility, autonomy, and the elimination of long commutes. Yet these same advantages come with hidden costs. Without the natural movement of commuting, the posture resets of hallway conversations, or the rhythm of leaving the office at day's end, our bodies and minds have lost many of the small recovery moments they once relied on.

The New Normal: Constant Connection

In today's knowledge economy, we often spend 8–12 hours a day seated, staring at screens. The line between "on" and "off" time is increasingly blurred. Many professionals find themselves responding to late-night messages, eating lunch at their desks, or skipping movement breaks altogether — a phenomenon some researchers now call *the urgency culture*.

While technology allows us to work anywhere, it also tempts us to work everywhere. The constant pull of notifications and digital tasks can overload the nervous system, leading to mental exhaustion that mirrors physical fatigue.

The body was not designed for this level of stillness or cognitive intensity. Without intentional recovery habits, the cumulative stress quietly manifests as tension, back pain, headaches, and disrupted sleep — all warning signs of an environment that no longer supports our biology.

Beyond Productivity: Redefining "Healthy Work"

For decades, wellness and productivity were treated as separate goals. Today, the science is clear: they are inseparable. Sustainable productivity depends on the body's ability to maintain energy, posture, and focus over time.

Ergonomics — once considered the domain of chair adjustments and desk heights — has evolved into something broader: *a daily practice of movement, alignment, and mindful recovery.* The modern definition of ergonomics is not just how we sit, but *how we live while we work.*

This means expanding our perspective from isolated posture fixes to holistic habits — ones that include hydration, eye health, emotional regulation, and daily rhythm. True home office wellness is built not on expensive furniture, but on consistent micro-habits that align body, mind, and environment.

The Hidden Costs of Convenience

The shift to home-based work has created what experts call the *convenience paradox*: as tasks become easier and faster, human bodies move less and recover poorly. The same convenience that saves time quietly erodes our resilience.

Long hours in static postures compress spinal discs and restrict circulation. Reduced daylight exposure affects circadian rhythm and sleep quality. Social isolation diminishes mental health. Over time, these small daily stresses compound into chronic musculoskeletal pain, cognitive fatigue, and burnout.

The solution is not to abandon remote work, but to evolve with it — to build wellness practices that match the realities of this new landscape.

The Opportunity: A Wellness Revolution at Home

Despite its challenges, the rise of remote work offers a unique opportunity: control. We now have unprecedented power to shape our work environments, our routines, and our rhythms.

In a traditional office, wellness initiatives depend on corporate culture and facilities. At home, we become our own ergonomics specialist — designing environments that truly support our health, focus, and creativity.

The *Home Office Wellness Guide* will show you how to do exactly that — combining ergonomic science, movement psychology, and nervous system health into a practical toolkit for a sustainable workday.

Key Takeaways

Remote work has reshaped not just *where* we work, but *how* our bodies and minds respond to work.

Constant connection and reduced movement create new physical and emotional stressors.

True ergonomics now includes posture, recovery, hydration, vision, and nervous system balance.

The home office is not just a workspace — it's a personal ecosystem for health and performance.

Looking Ahead

In the next chapter, we'll uncover *the hidden costs of sedentary work* — exploring how sitting, stillness, and screen exposure quietly alter the body's structure, energy, and resilience, and how small daily corrections can prevent long-term strain.

CHAPTER 2

THE HIDDEN COSTS OF SEDENTARY WORK

Why Stillness Is Silently Reshaping Our Health

For much of human history, movement was woven into survival. We walked, lifted, reached, and turned as part of everyday life. Today, most of us perform the same motions — typing, mousing, scrolling — for hours at a time. The modern workday has compressed physical variety into a narrow range of repetitive micro-movements.

Remote work, while efficient, has magnified this stillness. Without the incidental movement of commuting or walking to meetings, the average home-based professional now sits more than nine hours a day — longer than many long-haul flights. The result is a slow drift toward deconditioning that rarely feels dramatic but steadily undermines strength, circulation, and focus.

1. The "Modern Posture Epidemic"

Prolonged sitting changes the body's default posture. Hip flexors shorten, spinal muscles weaken, and the head subtly drifts forward in response to screens. These structural shifts increase strain on the lower back and neck and restrict breathing capacity.

Research links these adaptations to headaches, shoulder tension, and even mood changes. Poor posture doesn't just look uncomfortable — it alters how efficiently oxygen and energy reach the brain. Over time, the nervous system begins to interpret this low-grade strain as a form of chronic stress.

2. The Metabolic Cost of Stillness

Muscle activity is more than movement — it's metabolic signaling. When large muscle groups remain inactive, circulation slows and the body burns fewer calories, affecting insulin sensitivity and inflammation levels. Sitting for long, uninterrupted periods can reduce lower-limb blood flow by nearly half, contributing to fatigue and swollen legs.

Even light activity, such as two minutes of standing or walking every half hour, reactivates these pathways. The message: small movement bursts prevent large downstream consequences.

3. The Mental and Emotional Toll

The cognitive side of sedentary work is equally significant. Monotony, lack of variety, and screen fixation deplete dopamine and dull concentration. The brain thrives on sensory change — different postures, perspectives, and light exposures. When those inputs disappear, focus falters and stress hormones rise.

This is why long digital sessions can leave you mentally foggy even if you haven't moved a muscle. Physical movement is, in many ways, mental movement.

4. Early Warning Signs

Most professionals don't recognize the early stages of sedentary strain because symptoms are subtle:

Frequent fidgeting or shifting in the chair

Tightness in the neck or between shoulder blades

Afternoon fatigue despite adequate sleep

Restlessness or inability to focus after long meetings

These are the body's prompts to change position and re-oxygenate muscles. Ignoring them allows tension to accumulate until it becomes pain.

5. Building Awareness

The first step toward reversing the effects of stillness is noticing how static your day really is. Many people overestimate how often they move. Using a posture-tracking app, smartwatch, or even a sticky-note reminder can reveal long sitting stretches you didn't realize existed.

Awareness turns motion into medicine. Once you recognize the pattern, micro-movement breaks become natural rather than forced.

Key Takeaways

Sedentary work changes posture, circulation, and metabolism in subtle but significant ways.

Regular movement — even brief — interrupts this cascade of strain.

Early cues like tension and fatigue are opportunities to reset, not nuisances to ignore.

Restoring movement variety protects both physical and cognitive performance.

Looking Ahead

Now that you understand the hidden toll of stillness, the next step is to *design your environment* so that movement and good posture become effortless. In the following chapter, we'll explore **Ergonomics for Energy** — practical workspace adjustments that turn your desk into an ally, not an obstacle.

Chapter 3

Ergonomics For Energy

For readers who wish to explore workstation setup and posture in greater depth, see my earlier book, ***Home Office Handbook – Ergonomic Solutions for Back Pain****, which provides detailed guidance on ergonomic seating, sit-stand transitions, and posture troubleshooting. This current volume builds on those foundations, focusing on how ergonomics supports sustained energy, focus, and mental clarity throughout the day.*

How to Design a Workspace That Fuels Focus and Reduces Fatigue

An ergonomic workspace is more than a comfortable chair and a tidy desk — it's an environment that works *with* your body instead of against it. When the physical setup supports natural posture and balanced movement, energy flows more efficiently, concentration sharpens, and strain fades into the background.

The goal of ergonomics is not perfection but *alignment*: between your body, your tools, and the tasks you perform most often. Once this alignment is achieved, energy once wasted on tension and discomfort becomes available for creativity, problem-solving, and calm focus.

1. The Energy–Posture Connection

Posture is not a fixed position; it's a dynamic process of balance. Every moment your body subtly adjusts to gravity, screen distance, and keyboard reach. When the setup is off by even a few centimeters, muscles compensate, draining energy reserves throughout the day.

The key principle: **energy follows alignment.**
When your workstation encourages neutral posture — upright spine, relaxed shoulders, open hips — muscles require minimal effort to maintain position, leaving more energy for mental tasks.

2. The Foundations of an Ergonomic Setup

A healthy workspace balances comfort, reach, and visibility. Think of it as an ecosystem where each element influences the next.

Chair

Choose one with adjustable seat height, lumbar support, and a stable base.

Adjust height so your feet rest flat and knees are roughly level with hips.

Sit back fully against the backrest to support your lumbar curve — avoid perching forward.

Desk

Height should allow elbows to rest at roughly 90 degrees when typing.

If the desk is too high, raise your chair and use a footrest.

Keep the area beneath the desk clear so you can shift leg positions easily.

Monitor

The top of the screen should sit near eye level and an arm's length away.

Tilt slightly upward to reduce neck flexion.

If you use a laptop, add a stand and external keyboard to prevent hunching.

Keyboard and Mouse

Keep them close to your body to avoid overreaching.

Wrists should be neutral, not bent up or down.

Alternate mouse sides occasionally to balance strain.

Lighting

Use natural light where possible, positioning screens perpendicular to windows to minimize glare.

Avoid harsh overhead lighting; use soft, indirect lamps when needed.

For evening work, warm-toned light reduces blue-light exposure and eye fatigue.

3. Common Ergonomic Mistakes

Monitor too high → creates neck and eye strain.

Monitor too low → encourages forward head posture.

Chair too high → legs dangle, increasing pressure on back and behind knees.

Keyboard too far away → promotes rounded shoulders and stress on arms.

Fixed posture → even perfect alignment becomes strain when static.

Ergonomics is not about freezing into "good posture." It's about creating *the freedom to move* without discomfort.

4. Designing for Movement

The most effective workstations invite motion.

Use a sit-stand desk or simply alternate between chair and counter-height surfaces.

Place the printer, water bottle, or phone slightly out of reach to encourage micro-movement.

Consider a small foot rocker or active-sitting stool to maintain subtle motion during focus tasks.

Movement-friendly environments prevent the "energy slump" that comes from long static periods and keep circulation steady throughout the day.

5. Personalizing Your Space

Ergonomics is personal — no two bodies or work rhythms are identical. Take time to fine-tune:

Chair height vs. armrest level

Distance between screen and keyboard

Lighting that complements your eyes, not the room aesthetic

Every small adjustment is an act of self-care and self-awareness. When your environment supports you physically, your nervous system can downshift from tension to calm productivity.

6. Quick Ergonomic Checklist

Feet flat, knees at 90°

Hips slightly above knees

Monitor top at eye level

Elbows close to body, 90° bend

Wrists neutral

Shoulders relaxed

Every 30–45 minutes: change position

Key Takeaways

Ergonomics is about alignment and energy efficiency, not rigidity.

A balanced setup reduces tension and improves focus.

Small adjustments compound into measurable physical relief.

Your workspace should *invite* movement, not restrict it.

Looking Ahead

Now that your workspace supports you physically, it's time to address another key element of health and comfort: **your vision.** In the next chapter, we'll explore **Visual Ergonomics and Eye Health** — how to protect your eyes, manage light, and reduce digital strain in the modern workday.

Chapter 4

Visual Ergonomics And Eye Health

Protecting Your Vision in a Digital Workday

Your posture may be supported and your chair adjusted perfectly — yet one of the most overworked parts of your body still bears the daily strain of modern work: your eyes.
Every email, document, and video call depends on them, yet few people think of eye care as an ergonomic concern. In reality, visual comfort is integral to productivity, focus, and long-term health.

1. The Hidden Epidemic of Digital Eye Strain

The average office worker now spends more than 1,700 hours per year in front of a screen. This prolonged visual focus narrows the eye muscles' range of motion and drastically reduces blink rate — sometimes to less than half of what's normal.

This combination of concentrated focus, reduced blinking, and high screen brightness leads to a cluster of symptoms known as **Digital Eye Strain (DES)** or **Computer Vision Syndrome**:

Dry, gritty, or watery eyes

Blurred or double vision

Headaches behind the eyes or temples

Neck and shoulder tension from leaning forward

Difficulty refocusing between near and distant objects

These symptoms often appear subtle at first but compound over time, especially in poorly lit home environments.

2. How Screen Work Affects the Eyes

When you focus on a nearby object, the eye muscles contract and the lens thickens — a process called **accommodation**. Holding this contraction for long periods is like keeping any muscle tense: fatigue builds and focus falters.

Digital screens add extra stress by emitting blue light, which scatters more easily and causes glare, particularly in dim settings. This increases visual effort and may interfere with melatonin production, affecting sleep quality later in the evening.

Add to that unbalanced lighting — windows behind screens or harsh ceiling lights — and the result is a perfect storm of visual and postural stress.

3. Creating a Vision-Friendly Workspace

Visual ergonomics aims to balance **clarity, brightness, and distance**. Here are practical adjustments that make a powerful difference:

Monitor Setup

Place screens **at or just below eye level**, about an arm's length away.

If you use multiple screens, align their top edges and angle them gently inward.

Keep a neutral gaze; looking slightly downward is easier on the eyes than upward.

Lighting

Use **indirect natural light** where possible, positioning screens **perpendicular to windows** to minimize glare.

Avoid bright light sources directly behind or in front of the monitor.

Use **task lighting** for reading, and reduce overall brightness to match your screen.

Screen Settings

Adjust brightness so white backgrounds aren't harsh — they should match your paper or surroundings.

Increase text size slightly; small print increases strain.

Use night mode or blue-light filters after dusk.

4. The 20-20-20 Rule (and Beyond)

A simple but powerful principle:

Every 20 minutes, look at something 20 feet away for at least 20 seconds.

This resets eye focus, encourages blinking, and reduces tension.
For added benefit:

Blink fully 10 times before returning to work.

Stand, stretch, or walk a few steps during that break — your eyes and spine will thank you.

Use digital reminders or apps that gently prompt you to pause and refocus.

5. The Role of Hydration and Air Quality

Dry eyes are often worsened by **low humidity, air conditioning, or dehydration**.
Encourage tear production naturally by:

Staying hydrated throughout the day.

Keeping indoor humidity between 40–60%.

Blinking consciously during intense focus periods.

Positioning fans or vents away from your face.

Hydration supports not only eye comfort but overall circulation and energy regulation — a theme we'll explore in depth later in the book.

6. Beyond the Screen

Regular eye check-ups are essential, even for those with perfect vision.

Ask your optometrist about computer-specific lenses or coatings.

If you wear glasses, ensure the prescription suits your working distance, not just driving or reading range.

Include visual recovery in your wellness breaks — looking out a window, focusing on distant movement, or simply closing your eyes for a few deep breaths.

These habits restore ocular flexibility and reduce fatigue, improving both comfort and concentration.

Key Takeaways

Digital Eye Strain is a widespread yet preventable result of screen overuse.

Visual ergonomics begins with balanced lighting, correct monitor distance, and mindful breaks.

Hydration and environmental comfort are critical for eye health.

Protecting your vision protects your focus — your most valuable cognitive asset.

Looking Ahead

With your eyes and posture aligned, it's time to reconnect your body to its natural rhythm of movement. In the next chapter, we'll explore **Movement Throughout the Day** — how to keep energy flowing, prevent stiffness, and build vitality into your work routine.

Chapter 5

Movement Throughout The Day

Reclaiming Motion in a World Built for Sitting

Movement is the foundation of human health. Every system in the body — musculoskeletal, cardiovascular, digestive, and even cognitive — depends on regular motion to function efficiently. Yet modern work has quietly engineered movement out of our daily lives.

We commute sitting, work sitting, and relax sitting. The result is a body built for motion forced into stillness for most of the day. Over time, this mismatch creates fatigue, muscle imbalances, and the sense of being "tired but wired" — mentally exhausted, yet physically restless.

The solution is not marathon workouts or expensive equipment. It's **frequent, low-intensity movement woven into the fabric of your day**.

1. Why Movement Matters More Than Exercise

It's easy to assume that a single daily workout compensates for long hours of sitting. Unfortunately, research shows the opposite: even people who meet exercise guidelines experience negative health effects if they remain sedentary for much of the day.

The body doesn't only need *exercise*; it needs *motion variety*. Short bursts of stretching, standing, or walking re-activate circulation, refresh the nervous system, and improve concentration.

Think of your day as a sequence of movement snacks — small, frequent, restorative motions that sustain energy and focus.

2. The Physiology of Micro-Movement

When you change position, even slightly, you trigger:

Increased blood flow to muscles and brain

Activation of postural stabilizers that prevent back and neck pain

Improved oxygen delivery and waste removal

Reset of visual focus and mental clarity

These "micro-resets" counter the cumulative stress of stillness. Over time, they reduce discomfort, improve mood, and enhance performance.

3. The Ideal Movement Rhythm

The human body thrives on cycles — not constant motion, but regular alternation between effort and release.

A simple rhythm to follow:

Move for one to two minutes every 30–45 minutes of focused work.

Set subtle cues:

Stand during phone calls.

Stretch or roll shoulders while reading emails.

Walk to refill your water glass instead of keeping it at your desk.

Use a sit-stand desk or vary your seat height through the day.

These tiny adjustments compound into meaningful physiological change.

4. Desk-Friendly Movement Ideas

You don't need gym clothes or spare time — just intention. Here are practical movement resets for different parts of the day:

Morning Activation

Shoulder rolls (10 each direction)

Gentle spinal twists seated or standing

5 deep breaths expanding the ribs sideways

Slow head turns to release the neck

Midday Reboot

Stand and march in place for 60 seconds

Calf raises (10–15 reps)

Open-chest stretch (clasp hands behind back and lift slightly)

Side bends or standing hip circles

Wall angels to open shoulders, stretching tight muscles

Afternoon Reset

Seated figure-4 hip stretch

Wrist and finger extensions

20-second forward fold to decompress the spine

2-minute walk — even around the room

Each of these helps reset both the musculoskeletal and nervous systems, reducing the mental fatigue that builds up through the afternoon.

5. Active Sitting and Posture Variability

Even while seated, you can stay dynamic:

Use a small cushion or balance disc (wobble cushion) to subtly engage core muscles.

Shift weight from one sit bone to the other every few minutes.

Vary leg positions — cross, uncross, extend.

Keep the chair slightly reclined at intervals to offload spinal pressure.

Movement is not distraction; it's energy management.
Micro-movements prevent stiffness, keeping your mind alert without the crash that follows prolonged inactivity.

6. Integrating Movement Habits

Behavioral cues make consistency easier:

Visual cues: Place a sticky note saying "Move" near your monitor.

Time cues: Pair movement with existing habits (stand when you send an email).

Digital cues: Use reminders or smartwatch alerts to stretch, blink, or breathe.

Make it part of your identity: *"I'm someone who moves often."*
This shift from rule to self-image makes movement automatic, not another task on your to-do list.

7. Movement and Mental Clarity

Movement changes brain chemistry. Even light physical activity increases serotonin and dopamine, neurotransmitters that enhance motivation and focus.
A quick stretch break can improve memory, creativity, and decision-making far more effectively than pushing through fatigue.

Many people find their best ideas arise during walks, not while sitting at a desk. Movement literally shifts perspective — a reminder that body and brain function best when they move together.

Key Takeaways

Movement throughout the day is essential, not optional.

Micro-movements maintain circulation, focus, and posture integrity.

Regular, gentle resets outperform long, infrequent exercise bursts for health and performance.

Consistency and rhythm matter more than intensity.

Looking Ahead

Now that you've learned to weave motion into your workday, the next step is managing **energy and focus** — not by working harder, but by working *with* your body's natural rhythms.

In the next chapter, we'll explore **Energy Management Over Time Management** — how to align your tasks with your biological cycles for peak performance and better recovery.

Chapter 6

Energy Management Over Time Management

Working With Your Body's Natural Rhythms

For years, professionals have been taught to manage their **time** — to plan, schedule, and optimize every hour of the day. But the real key to sustained productivity isn't time at all. It's **energy**.

Time is fixed. Energy fluctuates.
The most successful, resilient people don't work longer; they work *in rhythm* — aligning their most demanding tasks with their highest energy periods and protecting recovery just as carefully as performance.

1. Understanding Your Body's Rhythms

Human energy operates in repeating cycles throughout the day. These patterns, called **ultradian rhythms**, last around 90–120 minutes. Each cycle includes:

A peak of alertness and focus

A gradual decline in mental energy

A recovery phase when the brain craves rest or movement

When we ignore these natural waves — forcing ourselves to push through dips with caffeine or multitasking — we drain the nervous system and accumulate stress hormones like cortisol and adrenaline. Over time, this erodes focus, motivation, and even immune function.

Learning to work *with* these rhythms rather than against them is one of the simplest ways to boost both performance and wellbeing.

2. Mapping Your Personal Energy Curve

Everyone has unique energy patterns. Some feel sharpest early in the morning; others peak mid-afternoon.
To discover yours:

Over three days, note your **energy level** each hour on a scale of 1–10.

Identify the **two daily peaks** (when you feel most focused) and **two dips** (when you feel sluggish).

Use this pattern to plan your workday.

Example:

7–9am

High

Creative tasks, writing, planning

10–11am

Moderate

Meetings or collaborative work

12–1pm

Low

Lunch, walk, stretch

2–3pm

Moderate

Follow-up or focused work

4–5pm

Dip

Review, light admin, prep for tomorrow

Once you understand your personal rhythm, you can stop fighting fatigue and start scheduling tasks when your body naturally supports them.

3. The Myth of Constant Productivity

We often treat work as a straight line: start in the morning, power through until evening.
But biology tells a different story — productivity is a **wave pattern**, alternating between focus and recovery.

Trying to maintain high concentration all day is like running a marathon at sprint pace. The key is *oscillation*: alternating between periods of effort and renewal. Short breaks aren't distractions; they're maintenance for your brain.

4. Recovery as a Productivity Tool

The brain consumes 20–25% of the body's total energy. It needs oxygen, glucose, and rest to sustain performance.

Regular microbreaks — even 1–2 minutes of stretching, breathing, or looking away from your screen — help reset neurotransmitters, clear mental fog, and restore creativity.

Every recovery habit you build protects long-term focus.
Try structuring your day around this rhythm:

90 minutes of deep work

10–15 minutes of active recovery

Repeat the cycle 3–4 times, then take a longer midday reset

This structure aligns with your body's natural ultradian rhythm, making productivity sustainable instead of exhausting.

5. Energy Leaks: Hidden Drains in Your Day

Even with good posture and movement habits, energy can leak through subtle sources of tension or overstimulation:

Notification overload: constant pings keep your nervous system in alert mode

Poor hydration: even mild dehydration reduces focus by up to 10%

Skipped meals: glucose dips trigger mental fatigue and irritability

Lack of daylight exposure: disrupts circadian rhythm and sleep quality

Identifying and closing these leaks is often more effective than adding new wellness habits.

6. Building an Energy-Supportive Routine

Use this simple structure to design your ideal day:

Morning: Start with natural light, hydration, and gentle movement.

First Work Block: Do your most mentally demanding task while energy is high.

Midday: Move, stretch, and eat nutrient-dense food.

Afternoon: Switch to creative or social work as energy stabilizes.

Evening: Downshift — dim lights, reduce screen use, and allow the nervous system to reset.

You'll soon notice that your best work happens *between* breaks, not in spite of them.

7. Reframing Productivity

Working in tune with energy cycles requires a mindset shift. Productivity is not measured by hours logged but by **energy applied with intention**. When you stop equating stillness with laziness and start valuing rest as recovery, you free yourself from guilt and burnout cycles.

Energy management is not indulgence — it's efficiency.
A rested brain thinks faster, solves problems creatively, and maintains posture and focus effortlessly.

Key Takeaways

Time management without energy awareness leads to burnout.

Your body follows ultradian cycles of focus and fatigue; plan work accordingly.

Short, active recovery breaks sustain performance and protect health.

Managing energy, not hours, is the foundation of sustainable productivity.

Looking Ahead

In the next chapter, we'll dive into a practical extension of this concept — **The Power of Microbreaks** — showing how brief, intentional pauses throughout your day can reset posture, mind, and nervous system, transforming your productivity from reactive to restorative.

Chapter 7

The Power Of Microbreaks

Small Pauses That Restore Energy, Focus, and Posture

In a world that rewards constant activity, the idea of *doing nothing* for a few minutes can feel almost rebellious. Yet neuroscience shows that **short, intentional pauses** — microbreaks — are among the most effective ways to restore focus, reduce tension, and sustain energy across a long workday.

Microbreaks are not interruptions. They're **strategic resets** that allow your body and brain to recharge before fatigue and stiffness take hold. Think of them as "maintenance for your mind and muscles."

1. Why Microbreaks Matter

Every task, from typing to problem-solving, drains attention and physical energy. Without recovery periods, the nervous system remains in a low-level state of tension. This cumulative strain leads to fatigue, irritability, and the creeping discomfort that erodes posture over time.

Research shows that workers who take brief breaks every hour report:

Higher concentration and creativity

Reduced musculoskeletal pain

Lower perceived stress

Better decision-making accuracy

Even 30–60 seconds of mindful movement or breathing can lower muscle activation and recalibrate focus.

2. The Science of the Reset

The brain operates best in cycles of effort and rest — typically 90–120 minutes long (the **ultradian rhythm**).
Within these cycles, short pauses act as "micro recoveries" that prevent energy dips from deepening. Physiologically, a microbreak:

Increases blood flow and oxygen to the brain

Lowers sympathetic (stress) nervous system activity

Enhances vagal tone, supporting calm alertness

Reduces eye strain and muscle tension

When used consistently, these mini-pauses become a built-in nervous system training tool — helping your body recover faster and stay in balance.

3. What Makes a Break 'Micro'

A microbreak can be as short as **30 seconds** or as long as **3 minutes**. The goal is not to leave your desk for long periods but to **interrupt stillness** before it compounds.

A good microbreak has three qualities:

Movement - Changes posture or activates circulation

Breath - Slows the nervous system

Awareness – Shifts focus from digital to physical sensations

When these elements combine, the body resets — tension releases, focus sharpens, and energy stabilizes.

4. Practical Microbreak Ideas

Here are simple, evidence-based microbreaks you can rotate through your day:

Movement Breaks

Shoulder Blade Squeeze: Pull shoulders back and down, hold 5 seconds, repeat 5 times.

Neck Reset: Gently nod “yes” and “no” to release deep neck flexors.

Spinal Twist: Sit tall and rotate gently left and right.

Stand and Stretch: Reach arms overhead, then fold forward to decompress the spine.

Vision Breaks

20-20-20 Rule: Every 20 minutes, look 20 feet away for 20 seconds.

Blink Break: Close eyes and take three slow breaths to rehydrate the cornea.

Focus Shift: Alternate gaze between a near and distant object for 10 seconds.

Breathing Breaks

Box Breathing (4-4-4-4): Inhale 4, hold 4, exhale 4, hold 4.

Physiological Sigh: Two short inhales through the nose, one long exhale through the mouth.

Extended Exhale: Breathe out twice as long as you breathe in — calming the vagus nerve.

Mindful Breaks

Posture Check-In: Notice where your body holds tension; relax jaw and shoulders.

Mini Gratitude Pause: Name one thing going well today.

Grounding Moment: Feel your feet on the floor, notice your surroundings, breathe.

5. Frequency and Timing

The best schedule is **every 30–45 minutes**, or whenever you notice:

Eye strain

Shoulder or back stiffness

Diminished focus or irritability

You can set gentle cues — an hourly chime, a sticky note, or pairing microbreaks with natural pauses (like between calls or while files load). Over time, these breaks become instinctive rather than planned.

6. The Ripple Effect on Posture and Mood

Microbreaks do more than relieve physical strain. They **retrain the nervous system** to oscillate between activity and calm. Each pause teaches your body how to recover more efficiently, improving emotional regulation and mental resilience.

Consistent use of microbreaks also reinforces **postural awareness** — your sense of where the body is in space (proprioception). You begin to notice when tension starts building, allowing you to adjust before discomfort escalates.

As one researcher described it:

"Frequent microbreaks create a feedback loop — posture supports energy, energy supports focus, and focus supports posture."

7. Designing Your Microbreak Routine

Start small:

Choose **three types** (e.g., one movement, one vision, one breath).

Insert them into your morning, midday, and afternoon work blocks.

Gradually expand variety once it feels natural.

Example:

10:30 AM

Shoulder rolls + deep breath

Relieves upper back tension

1:00 PM

Stand, stretch, look outside

Boosts circulation & focus

3:30 PM

Physiological sigh

Reduces stress response

5:00 PM

Posture reset + gratitude pause

Marks transition out of work mode

In just a week, you'll notice improved posture, calmer energy, and fewer end-of-day aches.

Key Takeaways

Microbreaks are intentional pauses that prevent physical and mental fatigue.

Even 1–2 minutes of movement or breathing can restore focus and posture.

Consistency — not duration — drives results.

These small resets train the body to recover faster and work with energy, not against it.

Looking Ahead

Microbreaks are your first line of defense against stress and fatigue. But to sustain true calm and resilience, we need to understand the deeper system that regulates recovery — the **vagus nerve.**
In the next chapter, we'll explore **Vagal Stress Regulation** — how your

nervous system responds to work pressure and how to activate the body's built-in calming mechanisms.

Chapter 8

Vagal Stress Regulation

How to Activate the Body's Built-In Calm

Every time you pause to breathe deeply, stretch, or reset your posture, you're doing more than relaxing — you're stimulating one of the most powerful regulatory systems in the body: the **vagus nerve**.
This long, wandering nerve connects the brain to nearly every organ, forming the backbone of your **parasympathetic nervous system** — the part responsible for rest, recovery, and balance.

Understanding how to support this system can transform not only how you handle stress, but how you think, digest, and recover from a long day's work.

1. The Science of the Vagus Nerve

The word *vagus* means "wandering" in Latin — an apt description for a nerve that travels from the brainstem through the neck, chest, and abdomen, touching the heart, lungs, and digestive tract.
Its role is to keep the body's internal state in balance: slowing heart rate, promoting digestion, and lowering inflammation after stress.

When vagal activity is high, the body enters a state of **calm alertness** — focused but relaxed.

When it's low, the body remains in "fight or flight" mode, where tension, shallow breathing, and fatigue accumulate.

In modern life, constant digital demands and mental pressure keep many professionals unknowingly locked in low-vagal tone — chronically activated, yet depleted.

2. Vagal Tone: The Measure of Resilience

Vagal tone refers to how responsive your vagus nerve is.
High vagal tone means your body can switch easily between stress and recovery; low tone means it stays stuck in overdrive.

Signs of healthy vagal regulation include:

Steady, moderate heart rate

Calm breathing

Good digestion

Emotional steadiness

Signs of low vagal tone include:

Rapid or shallow breathing

Cold hands and feet

Digestive issues or bloating

Feeling tense even at rest

Improving vagal tone isn't complicated — it's about restoring natural rhythms of **breath, movement, and relaxation**.

3. Breath: The Fastest Way to Activate the Vagus Nerve

Breathing is the one automatic function you can consciously control — a direct doorway into the nervous system.
Slow, rhythmic breathing increases vagal activity by stimulating stretch receptors in the lungs and diaphragm.

Try these evidence-based techniques:

The 4-7-8 Breath

Inhale through the nose for 4 counts

Hold for 7 counts

Exhale slowly through the mouth for 8 counts
Repeat 3–5 times to lower heart rate and muscle tension.

Physiological Sigh

Two short inhales through the nose, followed by one long exhale through the mouth.
This pattern releases carbon dioxide and instantly down-regulates stress signals.

Extended Exhale

Make your exhale twice as long as your inhale.
For example, in for 3 seconds, out for 6.
Longer exhalations increase vagal tone and calm the body's internal rhythm.

4. Movement and Posture for Vagal Support

Gentle movement — especially with coordinated breathing — stimulates vagal pathways in the chest and abdomen.
Simple daily actions can make a measurable difference:

Seated spinal twists and chest-opening stretches

Gentle neck rolls to release tension around the vagus pathway

Light humming or singing to vibrate the vagus nerve through the throat

Regular walking outdoors, which naturally synchronizes breath and heart rhythm

Even your posture influences vagal activation.
When the spine is upright and the ribcage open, breathing deepens naturally — sending steady feedback to the brain that you are safe, not under threat.

5. Cold Exposure and Light Stimulation

Short bursts of cold water on the face or neck activate the vagus nerve through receptors linked to the "diving reflex."
Try finishing your morning shower with 10 seconds of cool water, or simply rinse your face with cold water when feeling stressed.

Similarly, morning exposure to **natural light** helps regulate circadian rhythm and supports the vagus nerve through hormonal balance and improved mood.

6. Social Connection and Gratitude

The vagus nerve also governs our **social engagement system** — the subtle network of facial muscles, vocal tone, and emotional resonance that enables connection.

Acts of kindness, laughter, and gratitude all strengthen vagal tone by shifting the body toward safety and trust.

Simple daily practices:

Smile intentionally — it triggers vagal pathways around the eyes and mouth.

Speak or sing softly to calm your breath and vocal cords.

Write down one moment of appreciation each evening.

Connection is biology's natural antidote to stress.

7. Integrating Vagal Regulation Into Your Day

You don't need long meditation sessions to activate calm.
Layer these micro-habits into your workday:

One slow breathing cycle before opening emails.

A brief humming exhale after stressful meetings.

A short walk outside at lunch to reset the nervous system.

A gratitude reflection at the end of the day.

These cues signal safety and balance — teaching the body that recovery is always available, even in busy moments.

Key Takeaways

The vagus nerve is the body's main pathway for stress recovery and calm.

High vagal tone supports relaxation, heart rate, digestion, and emotional balance.

Slow breathing, gentle movement, light exposure, and gratitude all improve vagal function.

Small, consistent practices create long-term resilience.

Looking Ahead

Now that you understand how to activate your body's built-in calm, it's time to explore another vital element of health and energy balance: **hydration and nutrition.**

In the next chapter, we'll look at how staying hydrated — both at your desk and throughout your day — supports concentration, posture, and nervous system function.

Chapter 9

Hydration, Nutrition and Energy

You can have the perfect workstation, great posture, and a calm mind — yet still feel fatigued if your body is under-fueled or dehydrated. Hydration and nutrition form the foundation of focus, comfort, and endurance. They influence everything from spinal health and muscle function to mood and decision-making.

In short, **your performance at the desk begins long before you sit down.**

The Power of Hydration

The human body is about 60% water, and the brain nearly 75%. Even mild dehydration — as little as one or two percent of body weight — can reduce concentration, increase fatigue, and trigger headaches or eye strain.

Water is not just a nutrient; it's the transport system that keeps every organ functioning efficiently. Without enough, every system works harder.

Hydration and Focus

When fluid levels drop, the body releases stress hormones that narrow focus and heighten irritability. This mild stress response explains why dehydration can feel like anxiety or brain fog.

Adequate hydration supports steady blood flow to the brain, helping you stay alert, calm, and mentally clear — one of the simplest productivity tools available.

Hydration and Posture

Your spine also depends on hydration. The cartilage discs between vertebrae act like water-filled cushions that absorb pressure throughout the day.

Long sitting compresses these discs, squeezing out fluid and reducing flexibility. Regular hydration, paired with movement and standing breaks, helps them rehydrate — keeping your spine resilient and comfortable.

How Much Water Do You Need?

Most adults benefit from **30–35 mL of water per kilogram of body weight per day**, or roughly **2–2.5 litres** (8–10 cups).

Increase your intake in warm climates or when consuming caffeine, which increases water loss. A simple guide:

If you rarely feel thirsty and your urine is pale yellow, you're likely well hydrated.

Smart Hydration Habits

Hydration is a rhythm, not a task. Try these small but powerful routines:

Drink a full glass of water on waking — before coffee or emails.

Keep a water bottle visible at your desk.

Take a sip during every posture break or micro-movement.

Add natural flavours like lemon, cucumber, or mint.

Use reminders or a marked bottle to track intake.

Small visual and behavioural cues help make hydration effortless.

Electrolytes and Balance

Water works best with electrolytes like **sodium, potassium, and magnesium**, which help fluid move efficiently into cells.

Natural options include:

Coconut water

Fresh fruit and vegetables

A small pinch of sea salt in your water on hot days

Avoid sugary sports drinks designed for athletes — they're unnecessary for desk work and often counterproductive.

Nutrition for Sustained Energy

Hydration and nutrition go hand-in-hand. Skipping meals or relying on caffeine causes blood sugar swings that lead to tension and fatigue.

Support consistent energy and focus with balanced fuel:

Start with protein: eggs, yogurt, nuts, or smoothies.

Include healthy fats: avocado, seeds, olive oil.

Eat lighter lunches: avoid heavy meals that drain focus.

Snack smart: pair fruit or whole grains with protein.

A nourished body sustains posture naturally — energy crashes are often fuel issues, not just ergonomic ones.

Hydration and the Nervous System

Hydration supports the **vagus nerve**, which regulates recovery and stress balance. When the body is well hydrated, heart rate variability improves — a marker of resilience.

Dehydration, on the other hand, stiffens both muscles and mood.

In simple terms: **water steadies both body and mind.**

A Simple Daily Pattern

8:00 AM - One glass before coffee
10:00 AM - Sip during stretch break
12:30 PM - Glass with lunch
3:00 PM - Herbal tea or infused water
5:00 PM - Final glass before finishing work

These simple anchors turn hydration into a daily rhythm instead of an afterthought.

Key Takeaways

Even mild dehydration impairs focus, posture, and mood.

Hydration supports spinal health, mental clarity, and stress balance.

Combine hydration with light movement and mindful eating.

Consistent, balanced habits sustain both energy and wellbeing.

Hydration Habits Checklist

Simple daily practices to stay focused, energised, and aligned.

☒ Morning

☐ Drink a full glass of water before coffee or checking emails.

☐ Refill your bottle or carafe and keep it within arm's reach of your desk.

☒ Midday

☐ Take a hydration break every 60–90 minutes — stand, stretch, and sip.

☐ Add lemon, cucumber, or mint for natural flavour and variety.

☐ Include a glass of water with lunch to aid digestion and sustain focus.

☒ Afternoon

☐ Swap your third coffee for herbal tea or infused water.

☐ Notice your energy — if you feel tired, drink before reaching for caffeine.

☒ Evening

☐ Drink a glass of water before finishing work to prevent evening dehydration.

☐ Avoid excessive caffeine after 2 PM to protect sleep quality.

☒ Weekly Check-In

☐ Track hydration for one week to find your natural rhythm.

☐ Aim for 2–2.5 litres daily (more if in warm climates or using air conditioning).

☐ Check your cues: pale yellow urine and steady energy signal good hydration.

Remember: Hydration isn't a single action — it's a flow that supports every movement, thought, and moment of focus throughout your day.

CHAPTER 10

DIGITAL WELLNESS & TECHNOLOGY BOUNDARIES

Reclaiming Attention and Calm in a Hyperconnected World

Technology has transformed the way we work — and, increasingly, the way we rest. Our devices now serve as our office, meeting room, social hub, and source of news. While this connectivity brings remarkable convenience, it also creates an invisible load on the brain and body: constant alertness.

Digital wellness isn't about rejecting technology — it's about creating **healthy boundaries** so that technology supports your goals rather than dictates your state of mind.

1. The Attention Economy

Modern digital platforms are designed to compete for attention. Each notification, alert, and scrolling feed triggers small bursts of dopamine, the brain's reward chemical. Over time, this creates a subtle state of *hypervigilance* — the same biological mechanism once used to detect danger now keeps us checking our phones every few minutes.

The result? Fragmented focus, elevated stress hormones, and reduced ability to enter deep work or true rest. Even brief distractions — a single message or ping — can increase mental recovery time by up to 20 minutes.

2. The Cost of Constant Connectivity

Working from home blurs the line between "on" and "off." Without clear physical boundaries, the brain struggles to disengage. Common consequences include:

Difficulty concentrating on complex tasks

Mental fatigue or "digital hangover" by afternoon

Sleep disruption due to evening screen exposure

Reduced creativity from lack of mental quiet

Emotional exhaustion from information overload

Left unchecked, this always-on pattern mirrors chronic stress, keeping the nervous system in a low-grade fight-or-flight state — exactly what your ergonomic and hydration habits aim to prevent.

3. Understanding Digital Fatigue

Digital fatigue is more than eye strain. It's a full-body experience. Extended screen exposure reduces blinking, restricts breathing, and limits micro-movement — all of which reduce oxygen flow and increase tension.

You may notice subtle warning signs:

Tightness in the neck or jaw after online meetings

Irritability or distraction after heavy device use

Trouble “switching off” after work hours

Recognizing these cues is the first step toward regaining control of your digital environment.

4. Creating Healthy Digital Boundaries

The goal is not to disconnect completely but to **reintroduce balance** — moments of silence, stillness, and choice. Here are practical strategies to implement immediately:

Define Digital Start and Stop Times

Set a clear **“digital sunset”** — ideally one hour before bed — when work notifications end.

Avoid reaching for your phone within the first 30 minutes of waking; start with light, hydration, and breath instead.

Segment Work and Personal Tech Use

Separate work and leisure devices if possible (e.g., phone vs. laptop).

Use separate browser profiles or app folders for “Work” and “Home.”

Log out of work accounts after hours to reinforce mental closure.

Control Notifications

Turn off nonessential alerts; check messages in batches instead of reactively.

Use “Do Not Disturb” or Focus Modes during deep work blocks.

Silence background pings from social apps — constant micro-stimulation is energy-draining.

Digital Detox Microbreaks

Step away from screens for at least 5–10 minutes every 90 minutes.

Use that time to move, stretch, or look out a window to restore natural eye focus.

Schedule one **screen-free hour** each evening or on weekends to reconnect with the physical world.

5. Managing Screen Exposure and Blue Light

Blue light suppresses melatonin — the hormone that prepares the body for sleep. To minimize its impact:

Use **blue-light filters** or night mode after sunset.

Reduce screen brightness to match ambient light.

Prioritize natural daylight exposure during the day — it anchors your circadian rhythm.

Avoid screens in bed; replace the late-night scroll with reading or relaxation.

Good light hygiene restores deeper sleep, which in turn supports posture, focus, and mood the following day.

6. Protecting Cognitive Bandwidth

Every open tab, alert, and mental task competes for the same limited resource: cognitive bandwidth. Clearing digital clutter has the same effect as tidying a workspace — it frees up attention for what matters most.

Close unused browser tabs.

Organize files weekly.

Keep your desktop minimalist — visual order promotes mental clarity.

Use a single to-do system (digital or paper) instead of multiple scattered lists.

This intentional structure lowers decision fatigue, allowing the brain to perform in a more relaxed, efficient state.

7. Reconnecting With the Physical World

The antidote to digital overload is sensory grounding — reconnecting with real-world input:

Step outside and notice temperature, sound, and light.

Touch something textured — wood, fabric, plants — to reawaken tactile senses.

Practice mindful breathing without a device nearby.

Reclaim pauses between activities instead of filling them with scrolling.

These simple acts remind the nervous system that it's safe to slow down.

8. Digital Wellness as a Leadership Skill

For team leaders and professionals in high-demand roles, modeling healthy digital behavior has ripple effects. Respecting boundaries — such as avoiding late-night emails — fosters a culture of recovery and trust. Digital wellness isn't just personal health; it's **organizational ergonomics** — aligning work culture with human biology.

Key Takeaways

Constant digital stimulation keeps the nervous system in a state of alertness.

Managing screen exposure and notifications restores focus and calm.

Clear start/stop boundaries protect recovery and sleep quality.

Digital wellness supports both personal resilience and team culture.

Looking Ahead

With your physical, physiological, and digital systems now in balance, it's time to address the broader picture — how to harmonize **work and life** in a sustainable way. In the next chapter, we'll explore Sleep, Light and Circadian Rhythms - the relationship between light and your internal body clock, and how to optimize your sleep.

Chapter 11

Sleep, Light, and Circadian Rhythm

Restoring Natural Balance in a Digital World

Sleep is not simply the absence of wakefulness — it's the body's most powerful recovery process. It resets your posture, restores spinal hydration, regulates hormones, and consolidates memory. Yet in today's digital world, artificial light, late-night screen exposure, and irregular schedules have disrupted the natural rhythm that once guided our energy cycles.

Understanding and working *with* your circadian rhythm — your internal body clock — is one of the most effective ways to enhance both productivity and long-term health.

1. What Is the Circadian Rhythm?

Your circadian rhythm is a roughly 24-hour internal cycle that regulates sleep, alertness, hormone release, and body temperature. It's governed by the **suprachiasmatic nucleus** — a small cluster of neurons in the brain that responds primarily to light.

When light hits your eyes in the morning, it signals the brain to raise cortisol (for alertness) and suppress melatonin (the sleep hormone). As daylight fades, melatonin rises again, preparing the body for rest.

Disrupting this rhythm — through late-night screens, inconsistent sleep, or poor light exposure — confuses these signals, leaving you feeling tired during the day and restless at night.

2. The Ergonomics of Light

Light isn't just visual; it's biological. The type, timing, and intensity of light you experience directly affect energy, mood, and even posture.

Morning Light: Exposure to natural daylight within the first hour of waking anchors your circadian rhythm and boosts serotonin (which later converts to melatonin at night). If you work indoors, open curtains fully or step outside for a few minutes early in the day.

Daylight at Work: Position your desk near a window when possible. Natural light stabilizes mood and reduces eye strain. If natural light is limited, consider a **full-spectrum light** to simulate daylight and maintain alertness.

Evening Light: After sunset, reduce bright overhead lighting and avoid cool-blue screens. Use warmer tones — lamps, candles, or amber light bulbs — to cue the body that it's time to wind down.

3. Digital Light and Sleep Disruption

Screens emit short-wavelength blue light that delays melatonin release. Even 30 minutes of late-night exposure can shift the circadian rhythm by an hour or more.

To protect sleep quality:

Use “night mode” or blue-light filters after sunset.

Lower screen brightness to match the room’s ambient light.

Avoid screens for at least 30–60 minutes before bedtime.

Choose restful transitions — journaling, stretching, or reading on paper instead of scrolling.

This small adjustment can dramatically improve sleep depth and next-day energy.

4. Optimizing Sleep Ergonomics

Your sleeping environment functions like an overnight ergonomic reset — allowing the spine, muscles, and nervous system to recover. To enhance recovery:

Mattress: Choose medium firmness to support spinal alignment.

Pillow: Keep head and neck aligned with the rest of the spine (not flexed forward).

Temperature: Keep the room cool (around 18–20°C / 65–68°F) — the body naturally sleeps deeper in cooler environments.

Darkness: Use blackout curtains or an eye mask to protect melatonin release.

The goal is *neutral alignment and minimal stimulation* — a sensory calm that promotes full physical recovery.

5. Timing Matters: Aligning Sleep and Wake Cycles

Aim for consistent sleep and wake times, even on weekends. This strengthens the body's internal rhythm and makes it easier to fall asleep naturally. For most adults, 7–9 hours of quality sleep per night supports optimal recovery, concentration, and pain modulation.

If your schedule allows, expose yourself to bright morning light soon after waking and dim light an hour before bed — the body thrives on predictable contrast.

6. The Midday Reset

Your circadian rhythm naturally dips in alertness mid-afternoon (around 2–3 PM). Rather than fighting this slump with caffeine, use it intentionally:

Step away from screens.

Stretch, hydrate, or take a brief outdoor walk.

Use a 10–15 minute rest or "non-sleep deep rest" (NSDR) session.

These restorative pauses prevent mental fatigue and support consistent energy through the day.

7. Posture, Sleep, and Recovery

How you sleep affects your posture as much as how you sit. During sleep, spinal discs rehydrate, muscles lengthen, and micro-strains repair. Supporting this process means avoiding positions that compress the neck or lower back.

Best positions:

Side sleeping: with knees slightly bent and a pillow between them.

Back sleeping: with a small cushion under knees to maintain lumbar curve.

Avoid sleeping on your stomach — it twists the neck and stresses the lumbar spine.

8. The Light–Mood Connection

Consistent light exposure also regulates serotonin and dopamine — neurotransmitters tied to motivation and focus. Lack of daylight can contribute to fatigue and low mood, particularly in winter months. If you experience mid-season dips in motivation, light therapy lamps (used for 20–30 minutes each morning) can help restore balance and alertness.

9. Building a Healthy Sleep Routine

Try this simple nightly rhythm:

8:30 PM

Dim lights, disconnect from screens

Signal wind-down

9:00 PM

Light stretching or gentle breathwork

Release physical tension

9:30 PM

Read, reflect, or gratitude journaling

Quiet the mind

10:00 PM

Lights out

Align with natural sleep onset

This predictable pattern reinforces calm and supports the body's natural clock.

Key Takeaways

Circadian rhythm governs sleep, energy, mood, and focus.

Light exposure — especially morning sunlight — anchors biological balance.

Screen and blue-light management protect melatonin and sleep quality.

Ergonomic sleep setups restore spinal and nervous system health overnight.

Consistency in sleep timing is more powerful than duration alone.

Looking Ahead

When light, sleep, and rhythm are aligned, focus, energy, and mood naturally improve. The next step is to carry this balance into *how* we live and work — blending personal and professional wellbeing without burnout.

In the next chapter, we'll explore **Work–Life Integration in the Hybrid Era** — how to translate these rhythms into sustainable, real-world balance.

Chapter 12

Work-Life Integration In The Hybrid Era

Creating Balance, Boundaries, and Sustainable Routines

For many professionals, the home office began as a temporary solution — a response to global disruption. Yet years later, remote and hybrid work have become the new normal. This shift has redefined not only how we work, but *how we live.*

Without commutes, physical offices, or clear start and stop points, work has expanded to fill every available corner of time. The challenge today isn't productivity — it's **protection**: safeguarding space for rest, focus, and real life within an always-connected environment.

Work–life integration is not about achieving perfect balance every day. It's about designing rhythms that align with your energy, values, and health — allowing both work and life to support each other, rather than compete.

1. The Myth of Balance

The phrase "work–life balance" suggests a perfect 50/50 split, but life rarely cooperates with symmetry. Some weeks are heavy on deadlines; others allow recovery and creativity. The key is **integration** — blending professional and personal responsibilities in a way that's fluid but not chaotic.

Integration begins with awareness:

What energizes you?

What drains you?

What boundaries help you stay calm and effective?

By designing around these questions, you move from reaction to intention.

2. The Hidden Costs of Boundary Blur

Without the physical cues of an office, home-based professionals often find themselves "half-working" and "half-resting" all day — never fully switching off. This blurred boundary contributes to:

Difficulty concentrating

Increased screen time and musculoskeletal tension

Poor sleep and emotional fatigue

Reduced satisfaction in both work and home life

Your nervous system thrives on contrast — clear transitions between focused engagement and genuine relaxation. Integration means creating deliberate *edges* in the day.

3. Setting Physical and Psychological Boundaries

Boundaries aren't walls; they're **frames** that protect focus and recovery.

Physical Boundaries

Designate a specific work zone, even if it's a corner or desk.

Use sensory cues to mark "work mode" and "home mode" — lighting, music, or scent.

Store work tools out of sight at the end of the day to help your brain disengage.

Psychological Boundaries

Begin each workday with a short ritual — deep breath, stretch, or cup of tea — to signal mental readiness.

End the day with a closing ritual — gratitude note, tidy-up, or short walk — to reset.

Communicate availability clearly to colleagues and family to minimize unplanned interruptions.

These simple transitions tell your brain: *work is over; recovery can begin.*

4. Designing Rhythms That Support You

Your day has natural peaks and troughs of energy (see *Chapter 6 – Energy Management*). Align tasks accordingly:

Use morning clarity for focused or creative work.

Schedule meetings and collaboration mid-to-late morning.

Protect midday for nourishment, light movement, and hydration.

Shift to lighter administrative work in the afternoon.

By syncing with your natural energy curve, you'll find that both work and home tasks feel less effortful.

5. The Role of Recovery

In traditional offices, microbreaks and social chats offered natural recovery. In hybrid settings, these must be *intentional*. Incorporate:

Short walks outside after major tasks.

Mindful breathing or stretches between video calls.

A consistent bedtime routine that includes digital downshifting.

Recovery isn't a reward — it's part of your workflow. Think of it as the *exhale* that allows the next *inhale* of focus.

6. Managing Home Environment Triggers

The home is full of distractions — dishes, laundry, notifications, or family noise. Effective integration involves realistic management, not perfection:

Batch household tasks into short time blocks to avoid constant switching.

Use noise-cancelling headphones or soft background sound to maintain focus.

When possible, communicate shared quiet times with others at home.

Boundaries succeed when they're clear but compassionate — firm enough to protect work, flexible enough to respect relationships.

7. Reconnecting With Your Non-Work Identity

Remote work can subtly compress identity — turning every space into a workspace and every hour into "potential work time." Deliberately reconnect with the parts of you that exist outside professional output:

Engage in a creative hobby.

Spend time outdoors daily, even for 10 minutes.

Schedule social or family connection with the same importance as meetings.

Restoring a sense of *self beyond work* rebalances the nervous system and sustains motivation long term.

8. Integration, Not Imitation

Many remote workers try to replicate the office at home — fixed hours, back-to-back meetings, constant availability. But the home environment invites a different rhythm. True integration embraces flexibility:

Allow short breaks for movement or hydration.

Use ultradian rhythm awareness to plan deep work.

Recognize that being productive at home may look different — and that's okay.

Your home office can become a space of renewal, not just output.

Key Takeaways

Work–life integration replaces rigid balance with flexible structure.

Boundaries create safety for both focus and recovery.

Daily rhythms, not strict schedules, sustain long-term wellbeing.

Protecting your non-work identity restores energy and purpose.

Looking Ahead

You've now built strong foundations — posture, movement, hydration, recovery, and balance. In the next chapter, we'll look at **Combating Isolation and Building Connection** — practical ways to maintain social health, belonging, and teamwork in the hybrid world.

Chapter 13

Combating Isolation and Building Connection

Nurturing Belonging and Emotional Wellbeing in Remote Work

Ergonomic health extends beyond furniture, posture, and physical setup — it includes emotional alignment. One of the most profound shifts in modern work is the quiet rise of *social isolation*. While digital communication has made collaboration easier than ever, many professionals feel lonelier and more disconnected than they did in traditional workplaces.

This isolation doesn't just affect mood — it influences posture, breathing, and motivation. Humans are wired for connection, and the absence of real social cues can subtly affect both health and performance.

1. The Hidden Impact of Isolation

When we work alone for long periods, the nervous system loses many of the micro-signals that regulate social and emotional balance — eye contact, body language, tone of voice. Without these, the brain can misinterpret silence as rejection or uncertainty, triggering low-grade stress responses.

Over time, this can manifest as:

Reduced motivation or purpose

Difficulty switching off after work

Increased tension and shallow breathing

Postural collapse (shoulders rounded, energy low)

A sense of disconnection despite constant communication

Awareness is the first step toward rebuilding connection — both with others and with ourselves.

2. The Science of Social Health

Social connection is as vital to wellbeing as sleep, nutrition, or movement. Meaningful interaction releases oxytocin and endorphins, lowering stress hormones and promoting cardiovascular health. High-quality social contact also supports vagal tone — the same system you learned to regulate through breath and movement in *Chapter 8.*

In essence, human connection is not just emotional — it's *physiological self-care.*

3. Signs of Social Disconnection

In remote or hybrid work, isolation often creeps in gradually. Watch for these indicators:

You rely solely on email or chat, avoiding calls or video.

Days pass without real conversation or laughter.

You feel emotionally "flat" or disengaged from your team.

Small problems feel disproportionately stressful.

Recognizing these patterns allows you to take proactive steps to reconnect.

4. Building Connection at Work

True connection is built through authenticity and consistency — not frequency alone. Here are practical ways to rebuild social health within hybrid and remote teams:

Intentional Communication

Replace some written exchanges with short voice or video calls — tone and body language matter.

Begin meetings with a one-minute personal check-in, not just agenda items.

Encourage team rituals — virtual coffee breaks, small celebrations, or shared learning sessions.

Boundary-Based Availability

Stay responsive during core hours, but protect deep work blocks from chat interruptions.

Let colleagues know when you're offline to normalize healthy boundaries.

Human-Centric Leadership

If you lead others, prioritize empathy. A brief "How are you doing?" can mean more than a dozen performance updates. Psychological safety — the freedom to speak openly without fear — is the ergonomic equivalent of mental posture support.

5. Reconnecting Beyond Work

Isolation isn't solved entirely at the professional level — it also requires personal grounding.

Schedule real-world interactions: coffee with a friend, a class, or community volunteering.

Move your body in social settings — walking groups, yoga classes, or team sports combine physical and emotional wellness.

Reinvest in hobbies or creative outlets that foster flow and joy.

These aren't indulgences; they're structural supports for mental and physiological resilience.

6. The Role of Compassion and Self-Kindness

Working from home can amplify self-criticism — the feeling that you should be "doing more." Compassion resets that loop.

Try this micro-practice: place a hand on your chest, take a slow breath, and repeat silently, *"I'm doing my best right now."*

Self-compassion activates the same neural pathways as social reassurance, improving emotional regulation and physical relaxation.

7. Designing a Connection Routine

Just as you plan hydration or microbreaks, schedule moments of connection:

Morning

Quick message or check-in with a colleague

Builds belonging

Midday

Short walk or shared lunch (in person or virtual)

Combines movement & connection

Afternoon

Gratitude text or voice note to a friend

Boosts mood and empathy

Weekly

Team catch-up or hobby group

Prevents isolation from accumulating

Connection is not an afterthought — it's maintenance for emotional ergonomics.

8. Posture and Presence

Interestingly, posture both reflects and influences emotional connection. When we feel isolated, the chest and shoulders tend to close forward — a subtle "protective" stance. Practicing open postures (shoulders back, chest lifted, slow breathing) sends feedback to the brain that it's safe to engage, helping counter feelings of disconnection.

As the body opens, communication becomes more natural — you literally become more approachable and receptive.

Key Takeaways

Isolation is one of the hidden stressors of hybrid work.

Social connection directly supports physiological health and vagal tone.

Intentional, authentic communication builds belonging and reduces fatigue.

Self-compassion and posture awareness both strengthen emotional resilience.

Looking Ahead

Now that you've learned to nurture physical, emotional, and social well-being, the final piece is longevity — sustaining these habits over time.

In the next chapter, we'll explore **Sustainable Wellness Systems** — how to turn everything you've learned into daily routines and lifelong ergonomic resilience.

Chapter 14

Sustainable Wellness Systems

Turning Daily Habits Into Lifelong Health

Wellness doesn't come from any single posture correction, meal plan, or stretch routine. It's built from a series of *small, repeatable actions* that, over time, create a self-sustaining system of health.

Just like a good ergonomic setup supports your body automatically, sustainable wellness systems support your wellbeing without relying on willpower alone. The key is consistency, not perfection.

1. The Shift From Effort to System

Most people approach wellness with bursts of motivation — starting a new program or routine, then losing momentum. The real transformation happens when you shift from *trying harder* to *designing smarter.*

A **wellness system** is a structure that:

Makes the healthy choice the easiest choice

Embeds habits into natural daily cues

Adjusts flexibly when life changes

When routines become automatic, you free up mental energy for creativity, relationships, and growth.

2. The Three Pillars of a Sustainable System

Every lasting wellness approach is built on three foundations:

1. Structure

Set clear anchors for your day — hydration reminders, microbreaks, meal times, and light exposure patterns. These create rhythm and predictability, helping the nervous system stay calm and focused.

2. Flexibility

Allow variation based on energy, workload, or environment. Some days you may move more, others you may rest. The goal is adaptability, not rigidity — a system that bends without breaking.

3. Reflection

Regularly check in with how your body and mind feel. Ask: *What's working? What needs adjusting?* This self-awareness keeps your system alive and responsive rather than mechanical.

3. The Habit Loop

Each habit follows a simple neurological sequence:

Cue → Routine → Reward

Cue: a trigger (e.g., finishing a task or hearing a reminder tone)

Routine: the behavior (e.g., standing stretch or sip of water)

Reward: the benefit or pleasant sensation that reinforces it (e.g., clarity, relaxation)

By intentionally designing each loop, you make healthy behaviors self-reinforcing. For example:

Cue: Email sent → Routine: Shoulder roll + deep breath → Reward: mini-reset of focus.

Over time, your environment starts working *for* you instead of against you.

4. Designing Your Personal Wellness System

Create a one-page framework — your personal *Wellness Map* — based on these categories:

Movement:

1–2 minute stretch or stand

Every 45 min

Calendar reminder

Hydration:

1 glass of water

Morning, mid-morning, mid-afternoon

After coffee

Recovery:

4-7-8 breathing or short walk

Between meetings

Calendar gap

Digital Hygiene:

Phone on Do Not Disturb

Deep work blocks

Start of task

Sleep

No screens 1 hour before bed

Nightly:

"Digital sunset" alarm

This small framework acts like an ergonomic manual for your body and mind.

5. The Power of Environment Design

Willpower fades; environment endures. Shape your surroundings to make healthy behaviors automatic:

Keep a water bottle on your desk and a yoga mat within reach.

Use natural light near your workspace to maintain circadian balance.

Place a reminder or affirmation where you can see it — something that brings you back to calm posture and intention.

Even subtle cues, like a comfortable chair setup or soft music during breaks, reinforce long-term wellness effortlessly.

6. Habit Stacking for Ease

To embed new actions, pair them with existing habits — a technique known as *habit stacking.* For instance:

After I open my laptop → I take three deep breaths.

After I finish lunch → I take a short walk.

After my last meeting → I stretch for one minute.

By anchoring new behaviors to existing routines, you eliminate friction and make change sustainable.

7. Progress Over Perfection

Sustainability thrives on progress, not pressure. You'll have days when structure slips — deadlines, travel, family life — and that's okay. What matters is the return, not the lapse.

View every reset as part of the rhythm, not a setback. This mindset shift transforms wellness from a checklist into a lifestyle.

8. Tracking and Reflection

Small weekly reflections keep momentum alive:

What actions made me feel most energized?

Where did tension or fatigue creep in?

What will I adjust next week?

Journaling or digital tracking helps identify patterns over time — giving you the same feedback loop that ergonomic assessment provides for posture.

9. The Longevity Mindset

Sustainable wellness isn't just about surviving the workday — it's about aging well. Ergonomic habits protect joint mobility, cognitive sharpness, and energy into later life. When you build consistent systems today, you're not only preventing pain — you're *future-proofing your vitality.*

Every breath, stretch, and pause becomes an investment in decades of comfort and capacity.

Key Takeaways

Systems, not willpower, create sustainable wellness.

Anchor habits in daily cues to make them effortless.

Prioritize consistency and reflection over perfection.

Environment design is the most powerful lever for long-term success.

The goal isn't constant optimization — it's living and working in alignment with your body.

Final Reflection

You've learned how posture, movement, hydration, and rest interconnect — forming a holistic ecosystem of health. The *Home Office Wellness Guide* isn't just about working better; it's about **living better while you work**.

Wellness isn't a destination — it's a rhythm. When you move, rest, breathe, and connect with awareness, you create a self-sustaining system that keeps giving back every single day.

Conclusion - Your Ongoing Wellness Journey

Living the Principles Every Day

Wellness is not a fixed destination — it's a living process. Every posture adjustment, mindful breath, stretch break, or glass of water contributes to a system of care that supports you far beyond the workday.

Through this guide, you've built the foundations for physical comfort, mental clarity, and emotional balance in your home office and beyond. You've learned that small, consistent actions — not major overhauls — create the deepest change.

1. The Power of Awareness

The most valuable skill you've developed is *awareness*. Awareness of how you sit, breathe, move, hydrate, and think. With awareness comes choice — the ability to respond rather than react, to realign your body and energy before fatigue takes hold.

Each moment of noticing is a step toward mastery. You now have the tools to listen to your body's signals and make adjustments before discomfort becomes pain.

2. Your Environment as an Ally

Your home office is no longer just a workspace — it's a living ecosystem that supports health, focus, and calm. From your chair height to your lighting, from your digital habits to your daily rhythms, every element plays a part.

Remember: ergonomic wellness isn't about perfection — it's about creating an environment that works *with* you, not against you. Over time, these surroundings become silent partners in your wellbeing.

3. Small Actions, Lasting Change

The most enduring wellness transformations come from micro-habits:

Standing to stretch between tasks.

Drinking water regularly.

Taking short mindful pauses.

Logging off with clear boundaries. Each small act sends a message of respect — that your health and time matter.

The compounding effect of these choices reshapes not only your posture but your outlook on work and life.

4. Extending Wellness Beyond Work

The posture principles and ergonomic strategies you've learned apply everywhere:

In the car: Adjust seat depth, support the spine, and pause during long drives.

At home: Use supportive seating when reading or watching TV.

During travel: Move and stretch regularly to offset long periods of sitting.

In sleep: Align pillows and mattresses to keep the spine neutral.

By integrating these habits across your lifestyle, you'll maintain energy, mobility, and comfort through every season of life.

5. The Journey Continues

Your wellness story will keep evolving. There will be days when you forget to pause, skip your stretches, or lose track of balance — and that's completely normal. What matters is the return: coming back to center, one breath at a time.

Each time you reset, you reaffirm your commitment to living in alignment — not only with your work but with yourself.

You've built a toolkit for resilience: posture, movement, hydration, rest, and mindful presence. Together, they form a blueprint for health that can adapt with you through any phase of work or life.

A Final Thought

Your home office is where you create, connect, and contribute — but it's also where you can thrive. Let your workspace become a reflection of how you care for yourself: balanced, calm, and ready for what's next.

Every day offers a new opportunity to practice awareness, restore balance, and nurture strength from the inside out. Your journey toward wellness doesn't end here — it begins anew, every time you sit, move, and breathe with intention.

Chapter 15

Conclusion - Your Ongoing Wellness Journey

Living the Principles Every Day

Wellness is not a fixed destination — it's a living process. Every posture adjustment, mindful breath, stretch break, or glass of water contributes to a system of care that supports you far beyond the workday.

Through this guide, you've built the foundations for physical comfort, mental clarity, and emotional balance in your home office and beyond. You've learned that small, consistent actions — not major overhauls — create the deepest change.

1. The Power of Awareness

The most valuable skill you've developed is *awareness*. Awareness of how you sit, breathe, move, hydrate, and think. With awareness comes choice — the ability to respond rather than react, to realign your body and energy before fatigue takes hold.

Each moment of noticing is a step toward mastery. You now have the tools to listen to your body's signals and make adjustments before discomfort becomes pain.

2. Your Environment as an Ally

Your home office is no longer just a workspace — it's a living ecosystem that supports health, focus, and calm. From your chair height to your lighting, from your digital habits to your daily rhythms, every element plays a part.

Remember: ergonomic wellness isn't about perfection — it's about creating an environment that works *with* you, not against you. Over time, these surroundings become silent partners in your wellbeing.

3. Small Actions, Lasting Change

The most enduring wellness transformations come from micro-habits:

Standing to stretch between tasks.

Drinking water regularly.

Taking short mindful pauses.

Logging off with clear boundaries. Each small act sends a message of respect — that your health and time matter.

The compounding effect of these choices reshapes not only your posture but your outlook on work and life.

4. Extending Wellness Beyond Work

The posture principles and ergonomic strategies you've learned apply everywhere:

In the car: Adjust seat depth, support the spine, and pause during long drives.

At home: Use supportive seating when reading or watching TV.

During travel: Move and stretch regularly to offset long periods of sitting.

In sleep: Align pillows and mattresses to keep the spine neutral.

By integrating these habits across your lifestyle, you'll maintain energy, mobility, and comfort through every season of life.

5. The Journey Continues

Your wellness story will keep evolving. There will be days when you forget to pause, skip your stretches, or lose track of balance — and that's completely normal. What matters is the return: coming back to center, one breath at a time.

Each time you reset, you reaffirm your commitment to living in alignment — not only with your work but with yourself.

You've built a toolkit for resilience: posture, movement, hydration, rest, and mindful presence. Together, they form a blueprint for health that can adapt with you through any phase of work or life.

A Final Thought

Your home office is where you create, connect, and contribute — but it's also where you can thrive. Let your workspace become a reflection of how you care for yourself: balanced, calm, and ready for what's next.

Every day offers a new opportunity to practice awareness, restore balance, and nurture strength from the inside out. Your journey toward wellness doesn't end here — it begins anew, every time you sit, move, and breathe with intention.

Dr. Susan Jameson *Chiropractor & Ergonomic Health Educator*

Home Office Wellness Guide – Ergonomic Habits for a Healthier, More Productive Workday

Appendix A - The 30-Day Home Office Wellness Reset Plan

The 30-Day Home Office Wellness Reset Plan

Available as a free pdf download from

Better Back Solutions

Download Your Copy Today!

This 30-day plan is your bridge from reading to *doing.* Each week focuses on one theme, gradually layering habits so they become automatic. By the end of 30 days, you'll have built a sustainable rhythm for physical comfort, mental focus, and emotional balance — all from your home workspace.

Structure of the Plan

☒ **Morning Reset** – posture, breathing, and light exposure

☒ **Midday Reboot** – movement, hydration, and focus recovery

☒ **Evening Wind-Down** – digital boundaries, relaxation, and sleep hygiene

Each action takes **2–10 minutes** — quick enough to fit any schedule, but powerful in combination.

How to Use This Plan Each activity follows a simple **Time – Action – Purpose** structure: *when* to act, *what* to do, and *why* it matters. This three-step format helps you build awareness and consistency — turning small daily actions into lasting ergonomic habits that support comfort, focus, and energy.

Week 1 – Foundation and Awareness

"Awareness is the foundation of change."

Day 1 – Morning Reset

Morning: Gentle neck and shoulder stretches (1–2 minutes).

Purpose: Ease stiffness and align posture before starting work.

Midday: Stand, roll shoulders, and walk for 2 minutes.

Purpose: Release upper-body tension and boost circulation.

Evening: end of workday - screen-free breathing pause (5 minutes).

Purpose: Calm the nervous system and transition out of work.

Day 2 – Hydrate and Move

Morning: Drink a full glass of water on waking.

Purpose: Re-hydrate after sleep and energize metabolism.

Midday: Do 10 desk-side squats or calf raises.

Purpose: Activate large muscle groups and refresh focus.

Evening: Gentle side stretch while standing.

Purpose: Reduce tightness from sitting and aid digestion.

Day 3 – Posture Check

Morning: Adjust chair height and monitor position.

Purpose: Maintain neutral spine and reduce neck strain.

Midday: Take a 5-minute walk outside if possible.

Purpose: Light exposure and circulation boost.

Evening: Sit tall, practice 5 deep breaths with relaxed shoulders.

Purpose: Re-set alignment before rest.

Day 4 – Eye Care Focus

Morning: Apply the 20-20-20 rule (every 20 minutes, look 20 feet away for 20 seconds).

Midday: Blink breaks + stretch wrists.

Evening: Dim lighting one hour before bed.

Purpose: Reduce eye strain and support circadian rhythm.

Day 5 – Light & Movement Awareness

Morning: Open blinds or step outside for 2 minutes of daylight.

Purpose: Anchor your circadian rhythm and morning alertness.

Midday: Stand meeting or stretch check-in.

Purpose: Promote movement variety and posture change.

Evening: Screen-free wind-down.

Purpose: Encourage restful recovery.

Day 6 – Breathing and Focus

Morning: 3 deep breaths before checking email.

Midday: Box breathing (4-4-4-4 count) for 1 minute.

Evening: Slow exhalation breathing before bed.

Purpose: Steady focus, reduce stress, and balance energy.

Day 7 – Active Recovery Sunday

Morning: Go for a short walk or gentle stretch flow.

Midday: Hydrate and do light household movement.

Evening: Reflect on your week: *What habits felt best?*

Purpose: Build awareness and motivation for Week 2.

Week 2 – Strengthening Habits & Postural Awareness

"Consistency creates confidence — keep showing up for yourself."

Day 8 – Sit–Stand Balance

Morning: Alternate between sitting and standing every 30–45 minutes.

Purpose: Prevent stiffness and improve spinal alignment.

Midday: Stretch your hip flexors for 1–2 minutes.

Purpose: Counteract prolonged sitting.

Evening: Gentle side bends while standing.

Purpose: Keep the spine flexible and relaxed.

Day 9 – Core Activation

Morning: Engage your core while seated — 3 sets of 10 seconds.

Midday: Standing pelvic tilts or torso rotations.

Evening: 5 deep breaths focusing on posture awareness.

Purpose: Strengthen stability and posture support.

Day 10 – Mindful Movement Breaks

Morning: 5-minute stretch routine before logging on.

Midday: Stand for one call or meeting.

Evening: Light walk or gentle yoga.

Purpose: Build movement variety into your day.

Day 11 – Hydration Focus

Morning: Start with 500 ml of water.

Midday: Refill bottle before the afternoon session.

Evening: Herbal tea or water instead of a late-day coffee.

Purpose: Support energy, focus, and joint health.

Day 12 – Shoulder & Neck Reset

Morning: Shoulder rolls × 10, chin tucks × 5.

Midday: Wall angels or band pull-aparts.

Evening: Gentle neck stretch with deep exhale.

Purpose: Relieve upper-body tension and promote alignment.

Day 13 – Eye & Screen Care

Morning: Adjust monitor height and brightness.

Midday: 20-20-20 rule practice.

Evening: Blue-light filter on all devices.

Purpose: Reduce digital eye strain and improve focus.

Day 14 – Weekend Reset

Morning: Outdoor movement or sunlight exposure.

Midday: Organize workspace for the week ahead.

Evening: Reflect — one habit that felt easiest to keep?

Purpose: Build awareness and momentum.

Week 3 – Energy, Light, and Recovery

"Recharge your body before it demands rest."

Day 15 – Morning Light Exposure

Morning: Step outside within 30 minutes of waking.

Midday: Open windows for fresh air.

Evening: Dim lighting one hour before bed.

Purpose: Support circadian rhythm and focus.

Day 16 – Breathing for Energy

Morning: 3 slow belly breaths before work.

Midday: Box breathing (4-4-4-4 pattern).

Evening: Gentle exhalation focus.

Purpose: Calm stress and regulate energy flow.

Day 17 – Move More, Sit Less

Morning: 2-minute mobility warm-up.

Midday: Short walk during calls.

Evening: Stretch hips and hamstrings.

Purpose: Prevent fatigue and stiffness.

Day 18 – Digital Boundaries

Morning: Delay email and news for 15 minutes.

Midday: Silent notifications for 1 hour focus block.

Evening: Screen free dinner or wind-down.

Purpose: Reduce mental overload and restore attention.

Day 19 – Circulation Boost

Morning: Ankle circles × 10 each side.

Midday: Calf raises × 15.

Evening: Legs-up-the-wall stretch.

Purpose: Enhance blood flow and recovery.

Day 20 – Mind–Body Connection

Morning: Brief gratitude note or reflection.

Midday: 5 deep breaths with shoulder release.

Evening: Gentle body scan meditation.

Purpose: Improve awareness and relaxation.

Day 21 – Sunday Reflection

Morning: Leisure walk or stretch routine.

Midday: Review progress, adjust environment.

Evening: Plan 3 wellness intentions for Week 4.

Purpose: Reinforce consistency and motivation.

Week 4 – Integration and Renewal

"Your habits become your environment — nurture both."

Day 22 – Posture & Focus Review

Morning: Posture check: feet flat, shoulders relaxed.

Midday: Mini standing stretch break.

Evening: Reflect — what posture habit helped most?

Purpose: Strengthen awareness.

Day 23 – Hydration Rhythm

Morning: Water first, caffeine second.

Midday: Add electrolytes or herbal tea.

Evening: Final glass of water before bed.

Purpose: Maintain steady hydration energy.

Day 24 – Movement Challenge

Morning: 3 minutes of mobility (neck, shoulders, spine).

Midday: Stand for 10 minutes every hour.

Evening: 5 minute unwind stretch.

Purpose: Build endurance and flexibility.

Day 25 – Stress Release Reset

Morning: Brief breathing or mindfulness practice.

Midday: Step away from screens and look outside.

Evening: Journal one positive shift you've noticed.

Purpose: Reduce tension and enhance mindset.

Day 26 – Eye & Wrist Recovery

Morning: Palming (cover eyes for 30 seconds).

Midday: Wrist rolls and finger stretches.

Evening: Gentle shoulder rotation.

Purpose: Prevent strain from screen work.

Day 27 – Environment Refresh

Morning: Tidy workspace or adjust lighting.

Midday: Add a plant or photo that inspires calm.

Evening: Quick gratitude reflection.

Purpose: Create a supportive, uplifting workspace.

Day 28 – Integrate & Sustain

Morning: Choose your favorite 3 daily resets.

Midday: Practice them mindfully.

Evening: Reflect on progress and energy levels.

Purpose: Consolidate new habits.

Week 5 – Completion & Forward Momentum

"Wellness isn't an endpoint — it's a rhythm you choose every day."

Day 29 – Personalize Your Plan

Morning: Note which resets you'll continue daily.

Midday: Schedule reminders for posture or breaks.

Evening: Relaxation routine of your choice.

Purpose: Build autonomy and self-motivation.

Day 30 – Celebration & Reflection

Morning: Celebrate consistency — acknowledge your effort.

Midday: Move, stretch, or take a mindful walk.

Evening: Write down 3 ways your body feels better.

Purpose: Reinforce progress and long-term commitment.

Weekly Reflection Questions

At the end of each week, jot a few notes:

What felt easiest to maintain?

What improved my focus or comfort the most?

Which habit needs a stronger cue or reminder?

How does my body feel compared to Day 1?

Reflection turns actions into insight — and insight into sustainable change.

Continuing Beyond 30 Days

When you complete the reset, you'll have a personalized rhythm that suits your energy and workspace. From here:

Keep your favorite 3–5 habits as *daily anchors.*

Revisit this plan quarterly or after life transitions.

Add variety — new stretches, hydration goals, or screen-free rituals.

The goal is not a perfect routine, but an adaptable system that supports you year-round.

Remember: Every posture adjustment, breath, or mindful pause is a small act of +prevention and renewal. By practicing these micro-habits each day, you're not just improving your work life — you're creating a foundation for lifelong ergonomic wellbeing.

Appendix B: Scientific References and Recommended Reading

This guide draws upon ergonomic, physiological, and behavioral science research from leading health and occupational wellness organizations. The following references and resources provide deeper insight into topics discussed throughout the book.

Ergonomics and Musculoskeletal Health

American Chiropractic Association. *Posture and Ergonomics at Work.*

Buckle, P. & Devereux, J. (2002). *The Nature of Work-Related Neck and Upper Limb Musculoskeletal Disorders.* Applied Ergonomics.

Hedge, A. (Cornell University Ergonomics Lab). *Healthy Computing and Home Office Ergonomics.*

Straker, L., & Mathiassen, S. E. (2009). "Increased Physical Workload in Modern Office Work." *Ergonomics*, 52(10), 1215–1225.

Movement, Sedentary Behavior, and Energy

Hamilton, M. T., Healy, G. N., Dunstan, D. W. et al. (2008). "Too Little Exercise and Too Much Sitting: Inactivity Physiology and the Need for New Recommendations on Sedentary Behavior." *Current Cardiovascular Risk Reports.*

World Health Organization. *Global Action Plan on Physical Activity 2018–2030.*

Tremblay, M. S. et al. (2017). "Sedentary Behavior Research Network Terminology Consensus." *International Journal of Behavioral Nutrition and Physical Activity.*

Visual Ergonomics and Digital Eye Strain

American Optometric Association. *Computer Vision Syndrome (Digital Eye Strain).*

Sheppard, A. L. & Wolffsohn, J. S. (2018). "Digital Eye Strain: Prevalence, Measurement and Amelioration." *BMJ Open Ophthalmology.*

Vagal Nerve Regulation, Stress, and Breathing

Porges, S. W. (2011). *The Polyvagal Theory: Neurophysiological Foundations of Emotions, Attachment, Communication, and Self-Regulation.*

Lehrer, P. M. & Gevirtz, R. (2014). "Heart Rate Variability Biofeedback: How and Why Does It Work?" *Frontiers in Psychology.*

Huberman, A. D. (2023). *The Science of Breathing and the Nervous System.* Huberman Lab Podcast & Stanford Neuroscience Institute resources.

Circadian Rhythms and Light Exposure

Czeisler, C. A. et al. (2019). "The Role of Light in Human Circadian Physiology." *Nature Reviews Neuroscience.*

Harvard Medical School. *Blue Light Has a Dark Side.*

Lockley, S. W. (2015). "Circadian Rhythms and Sleep in the Modern Workplace." *Occupational Medicine.*

Workplace Wellness and Behavior Change

Deci, E. L. & Ryan, R. M. (2000). "Self-Determination Theory and the Facilitation of Intrinsic Motivation." *American Psychologist.*

World Health Organization. *Healthy Workplaces Framework and Model.*

American Psychological Association. *Stress in America: Work and Well-Being.*

Appendix C - Recommended Apps, Devices & Resources (USA Edition)

Tools to Support a Healthier, More Productive Workday

The purpose of this appendix is to help you translate ergonomic principles into daily practice using simple, reliable tools. These apps and devices are selected for their accessibility and evidence-based design. Choose the ones that best fit your personal needs and working style.

⊠ 1. Posture and Ergonomic Support Devices

Smart posture tools and adjustable equipment can make it easier to maintain healthy alignment and reduce fatigue.

Sit–stand desk converters

Fully Jarvis • VariDesk • FlexiSpot

Alternate between sitting and standing to boost circulation and posture.

Ergonomic chairs

Herman Miller Aeron • NeueChair • Sihoo M57

Support the lumbar curve and reduce static load.

Footrests

Humanscale Foot Machine • Kensington SoleMate

Promote circulation and spinal balance.

Monitor risers / arms

Ergotron LX • Amazon Basics Adjustable Arm

Keep screens at eye level to reduce neck strain.

Keyboard & mouse alternatives

Logitech Ergo K860 • Anker Vertical Mouse

Encourage neutral wrist and forearm position.

Smart posture trainers

Upright GO • Lumo Lift

Provide gentle vibration reminders to correct slouching.

⊠ 2. Movement, Stretch, and Exercise Apps

Movement reminders and short guided routines help offset long sitting hours.

Stretch reminders

Stretchly • Move • Workrave

Custom microbreak prompts with timing flexibility.

Guided mobility

Down Dog • Yoga for Beginners • StretchIt

Short, posture-friendly mobility sessions.

Activity pacing

Pomofocus • Time Out

Combine work focus blocks with movement breaks.

Breathing and relaxation

Calm • Headspace • Breathwrk

Structured breathwork to calm and refocus.

☒ 3. Hydration and Nutrition Support

Hydration apps and connected bottles provide gentle cues to maintain optimal fluid intake.

Hydration reminder apps

WaterMinder • Plant Nanny • Aqualert

Track intake and send reminders.

Smart water bottles

HidrateSpark • Thermos Connected

Record consumption and sync to mobile devices.

Healthy recipe & meal prep

Lifesum • MyFitnessPal • Yazio

Balance energy, hydration, and nutrient intake.

☒ 4. Light and Circadian Rhythm Tools

Light exposure profoundly affects alertness and recovery. Use these to balance natural rhythms.

Blue-light filters

f.lux • Iris • Night Shift • Windows Night Light

Reduce evening blue light to protect melatonin.

Daylight simulators

Philips Wake-Up Light • Lumie Bodyclock

Support morning energy and circadian stability.

Sleep tracking

Oura Ring • Sleep Cycle • Fitbit

Monitor sleep duration and quality trends.

☒ 5. Digital Wellness and Focus Apps

These help you protect attention and prevent digital overload.

Distraction blockers

Freedom • FocusMe • Cold Turkey

Limit app or web access during focus periods.

Productivity & planning

Notion • Todoist • Sunsama

Organize deep-work blocks and rest intervals.

Digital detox tools

Forest • OffScreen • One Sec

Reinforce intentional phone and screen use.

⊠ 6. Mind–Body and Stress Regulation

Support vagal tone and recovery through mindful technology.

Biofeedback devices

HeartMath Inner Balance • Core Meditation Trainer

Train HRV and stress recovery awareness.

Meditation apps

Insight Timer • Balance • Calm

Build daily mindfulness routines.

Gratitude / journaling

Presently • Five Minute Journal • Stoic

Cultivate positivity and reflective awareness.

☒ 7. Trusted Resources for Continued Learning

Explore these reputable sources for ergonomics and wellness guidance.

OSHA – Ergonomics

Practical guidelines for office and remote workers.

Human Factors & Ergonomics Society (HFES)

Research and best practice updates.

Mayo Clinic – Posture & Ergonomics

Clear, patient-focused advice on body mechanics.

Sleep Foundation – Circadian Health

Evidence-based sleep hygiene education.

NIOSH – Workplace Health & Safety

Ongoing research into occupational wellbeing.

Final Note

Technology should **enhance awareness**, not replace it.
Choose tools that make healthy habits easier, not more complicated.
Let each device or app become a small reminder to pause, move, and realign — both physically and mentally.

APPENDIX D - RECOMMENDED APPS, DEVICES & RESOURCES (UK EDITION)

Tools to Support a Healthier, More Productive Workday

The following tools, devices, and resources can help you build ergonomic awareness and sustain energy throughout your day. Each one has been chosen for reliability, accessibility, and availability in the UK. Select those that best fit your working style and goals.

☒ 1. Posture and Ergonomic Support Devices

Smart posture tools and adjustable furniture make it easier to maintain alignment and reduce fatigue.

Sit–stand desk converters

FlexiSpot UK, Yo-Yo Desk, Fully Jarvis

Amazon.co.uk • Posturite.co.uk

Alternate positions to boost circulation and focus.

Ergonomic chairs

Herman Miller Sayl, Sihoo M18, ErgoChair UK

John Lewis • Posturite • Amazon.co.uk

Support lumbar curve and long-term comfort.

Footrests

Fellowes Professional, Kensington SoleMate

Argos • Amazon.co.uk

Improve circulation and promote spinal balance.

Monitor risers / arms

VonHaus Adjustable Arm, Ergotron LX

Amazon.co.uk • Ryman

Keep screens at eye level to reduce neck strain.

Keyboard & mouse alternatives

Logitech Ergo K860, Anker Vertical Mouse

Amazon.co.uk

Encourage neutral wrist and shoulder alignment.

Smart posture trainers

Upright GO 2, Lumo Lift

Amazon.co.uk

Gentle vibration reminders to correct slouching.

⊠ 2. Movement, Stretch, and Exercise Apps

Micro-movement breaks and mobility prompts help offset long sitting hours.

Stretchly – Customisable desktop break reminders.

Move or Workrave – Encourages frequent posture resets.

Yoga for Beginners or StretchIt – Guided, short-format mobility sessions.

Pomofocus – Combines focus blocks with movement prompts.

Breathwrk or Headspace – Short breathing or mindfulness exercises.

⊠ 3. Hydration and Nutrition Support

Keeping hydration steady supports energy, concentration, and joint health.

WaterMinder or Aqualert – Hydration reminders and tracking.

HidrateSpark – Smart bottle that tracks intake via Bluetooth.

Lifesum, MyFitnessPal, or Yazio – Balanced meal tracking and nutrition awareness.

NHS Better Health – Eat Well Programme – Reliable national nutrition advice.

⊠ 4. Light and Circadian Rhythm Tools

Light exposure affects alertness and recovery. Use these tools to align your body clock.

f.lux, Iris, or Night Shift (Mac) – Reduce evening blue light.

Lumie Bodyclock or Philips Wake-Up Light – Simulate dawn and support morning energy.

Sleep Cycle or Fitbit – Monitor sleep duration and quality trends.

The Sleep Charity UK – Expert tips on light, rest, and recovery.

⊠ 5. Digital Wellness and Focus Apps

Protect focus, reduce distraction, and manage digital boundaries.

Freedom or FocusMe – Block apps or websites during focus periods.

Notion, Todoist, or Sunsama – Organise priorities and task flow.

Forest or OffScreen – Encourage intentional phone use.

MindTools Stress Management – UK resource for balanced productivity.

⊠ 6. Mind–Body and Stress Regulation

Encourage mindfulness, breathing, and emotional resilience.

Calm, Insight Timer, or Balance – Guided meditation and relaxation.

HeartMath Inner Balance – Biofeedback for heart-rate variability training.

Five Minute Journal App – Daily gratitude and reflection prompts.

Mind UK – Trusted mental-health charity offering workplace wellbeing resources.

⊠ 7. Trusted Resources for Further Reading (UK)

HSE (Health and Safety Executive) – *Display Screen Equipment (DSE) Guidance*

Legal and practical standards for safe home workstations.

NHS Live Well – Working from Home

Evidence-based advice on posture, breaks, and routine.

The Sleep Charity UK

National guidance on rest, rhythm, and sleep hygiene.

Chartered Institute of Ergonomics and Human Factors (CIEHF)

Research and practitioner resources in ergonomics.

Mind UK – Workplace Wellbeing

Practical strategies for mental health at work.

Final Note

Technology and tools should enhance awareness — not replace it.
Choose resources that make healthy habits easier, not more complicated.
Let each one serve as a gentle cue to move, pause, and realign — both physically and mentally.

Appendix E - Recommended Apps, Devices & Resources (Australia Edition)

Tools to Support a Healthier, More Productive Workday

This list highlights reliable ergonomic tools, devices, and wellness resources available in Australia. Each one supports posture, comfort, and energy for remote or hybrid work environments.

⊠ 1. Posture and Ergonomic Support Devices

Smart ergonomic furniture and posture tools can make daily work more comfortable and sustainable.

Sit–stand desk converters

Ergotron WorkFit, OMNIDESK AU, Zen Space Desks

Officeworks • Ergolink • Amazon.com.au

Alternate between sitting and standing to improve circulation and focus.

Ergonomic chairs

Humanscale Freedom, Herman Miller Aeron, ErgoTune Supreme

Temple & Webster • Ergolink • Elite Office Furniture

Support lumbar curve and reduce long-term back strain.

Footrests

Kensington SoleMate, Fellowes Professional

Officeworks • Amazon.com.au

Improve lower-body circulation and posture.

Monitor risers / arms

Ergotron LX, Brateck, Vision Mounts

Officeworks • Amazon.com.au

Keep screens at eye level to reduce neck strain.

Keyboard & mouse alternatives

Logitech Ergo K860, Anker Vertical Mouse, Microsoft Sculpt Ergonomic Set

JB Hi-Fi • Officeworks • Amazon.com.au

Maintain natural wrist and forearm alignment.

Smart posture trainers

Upright GO 2, Lumo Lift

Amazon.com.au

Provide gentle reminders to maintain good posture.

⊠ 2. Movement, Stretch, and Exercise Apps

Movement breaks and guided mobility sessions help offset long sitting hours.

Stretchly or Move – Automatic microbreak reminders.

Down Dog or StretchIt – Short mobility or yoga routines.

Pomofocus or Time Out – Combine work intervals with active breaks.

Smiling Mind (Australian mindfulness app) – Guided focus and breathing.

Headspace or Calm – Relaxation and mental reset tools.

⊠ 3. Hydration and Nutrition Support

Staying hydrated supports focus, energy, and spinal health.

WaterMinder or Aqualert – Hydration tracking apps.

HidrateSpark – Bluetooth-enabled smart water bottles.

Lifesum or MyFitnessPal – Nutrition and meal tracking.

Healthy Eating Advisory Service (VIC Gov) – Practical nutrition and work-place wellness advice.

Eat for Health (Australian Government) – National dietary guidelines.

⊠ 4. Light and Circadian Rhythm Tools

Balanced light exposure improves energy and sleep quality.

f.lux, Iris, or Night Shift – Reduce blue light from screens in the evening.

Philips SmartSleep or Lumie Bodyclock – Simulate sunrise to support wake rhythm.

Fitbit or Oura Ring – Track sleep duration and recovery trends.

Sleep Health Foundation (Australia) – Reliable educational resources on light and rest.

⊠ 5. Digital Wellness and Focus Apps

Manage screen time, focus, and productivity intentionally.

Freedom or FocusMe – Block distractions to improve deep work.

Notion, Todoist, or Trello – Organise priorities and project flow.

Forest or OffScreen – Help maintain mindful phone habits.

Beyond Blue – Resources for managing stress and mental wellbeing.

⊠ 6. Mind–Body and Stress Regulation

Support mental balance, calm, and recovery throughout the day.

Smiling Mind – Free Australian mindfulness program.

Calm or Insight Timer – Meditation and breathing exercises.

HeartMath Inner Balance – Biofeedback and breathing for stress recovery.

Mindful in May (Australia) – Annual mindfulness challenge and community.

Black Dog Institute – Workplace mental health programs and tools.

☒ 7. Trusted Australian Resources for Further Reading

Safe Work Australia

National ergonomics and work health guidelines.

Australian Government – Comcare

Office ergonomics and injury prevention resources.

Sleep Health Foundation

Research and advice on healthy sleep and circadian rhythm.

Black Dog Institute

Evidence-based workplace mental health resources.

Smiling Mind

Free tools for mindfulness and focus at work.

OrganisationFocus

Final Note

Use technology to support awareness — not replace it. Choose tools and habits that make your day more balanced, your posture stronger, and your focus clearer. Small, consistent actions lead to lasting results.

Author

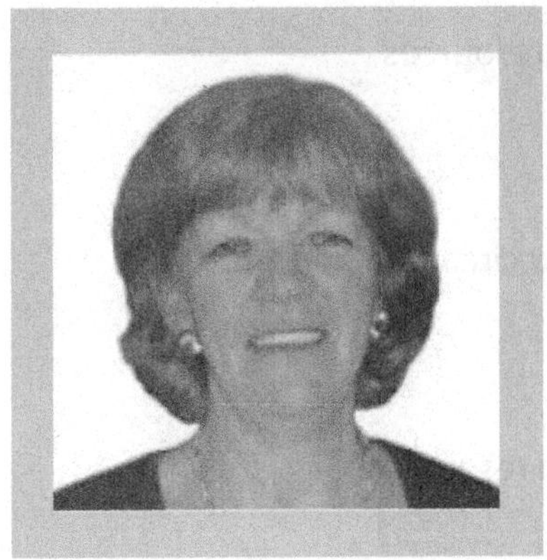

Dr Susan Jameson is a chiropractor, author, and ergonomics advocate dedicated to helping people work comfortably and live well. With more than forty years of clinical experience, she combines evidence-based ergonomics with simple daily practices that reduce pain, improve energy, and support long-term wellbeing.

She is the author of the *Ergonomic Wellness Series*, including:

• *Home Office Handbook – Ergonomic Solutions for Back Pain*

• *Home Office Wellness Guide – Ergonomic Habits for a Healthier, More Productive Workday*

• *Home Office Journal – A 30-Day Ergonomic Workbook*

Her work empowers readers to build healthier, more mindful relationships with how they sit, move, and work — one small adjustment at a time. Whether you're a professional, student, or freelancer, her practical guidance helps you feel better throughout your day.

Learn more at: https://betterbacksolutions.com.au

Also By This Author

Discover more titles in the Ergonomic Wellness Series

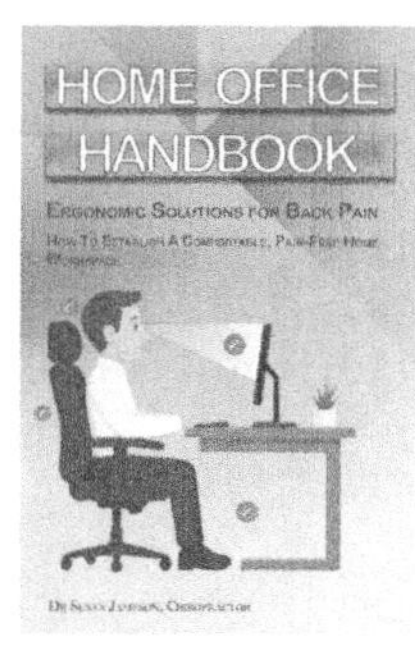

Home Office Handbook - Ergonomic Solutions For Back Pain

A practical, step-by-step guide to setting up your desk, improving posture, and reducing back, neck, and arm discomfort.

Scan the QR code to see this book at your preferred retailer

or visit https://books2read.com/u/mgB2oX

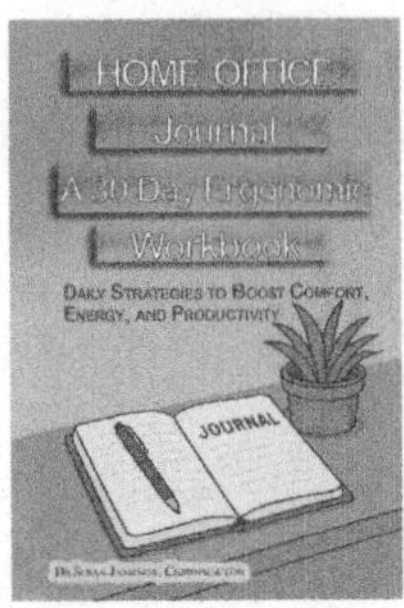

Home Office Journal – A 30-Day Ergonomic Workbook

Put ergonomic principles into practice with this 30-day workbook of daily prompts, checklists, and reflections designed to build healthier, more productive work habits.

Scan the QR code to see this book at your preferred retailer

or visit https://mybook.to/HomeOfficeJournal

LEAVE A REVIEW

If this guide helped make your workday more comfortable or productive, please consider leaving a short review at your preferred online book retailer.

Your feedback helps other readers discover the benefits of this book.

Thank you!

Scan the QR code to go to the book page

or visit:

https://books2read.com/u/4ADrWo

Made in the USA
Monee, IL
01 February 2026